ALLSPICE

MARIAN KIM

ISBN: 150856177X

ISBN-13: 978-1508561774

CONTENTS

MARIAN KIM

1

PROPERTIES

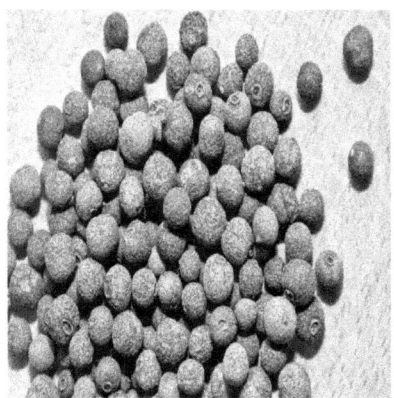

Scientific name: Pimenta dioica

Other names: Clove pepper, Jamaica pepper, water of pimento, myrtle pepper, newspice, pimento

Nutrients: Vitamins A, B1 (thiamine), B2 (riboflavin), B3 (niacin) and C. Minerals like iron, potassium, magnesium, selenium and manganese.

Properties

Carminative properties (prevents and relieves flatulence which is the formation of gas in the intestinal tract)

Antioxidant properties which protect the cells from free radical damage

Analgesic (pain relieving) properties

Antiseptic (antifungal) properties

Anti-depressant properties

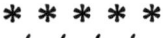

2

USES

Gas and bloating treatment

Allspice has carminative properties and allspice tea or allspice infusion can be consumed to treat intestinal gas. Allspice decoction can also be used to treat flatulence.

Indigestion treatment

Allspice is used to treat dyspepsia or indigestion. It is thought to stimulate the gastrointestinal tract's motility and the production of digestive enzymes. Allspice tea and allspice infusion are therefore consumed after meals to aid with digestion.

Diarrhea and vomiting treatment

Allspice is used to manage diarrhea, nausea and vomiting. It is also given for abdominal pain.

Anorexia treatment

Allspice is used to manage anorexia and improve the appetite.

Muscle pain relief

Allspice poultice is applied to the skin to relieve muscle pain. The poultice can be wrapped in a clean gauze to keep it in place and it should be left over the painful area for at least 20 minutes. Allspice salve can also be used for this purpose.

Joint pain relief

Allspice poultice are also used to relive the joint pains or arthritis and rheumatism. Allspice salve can also be used for this purpose.

Bruise treatment

Allspice poultice are used to treat bruises.

Depression management

Allspice is used to manage depression.

Heavy menstruation

Allspice is used by women with heavy menstrual periods and menstrual cramps.

Fever

Allspice is given to persons with fever.

Colds

Allspice is used to manage coughs, colds and the flu. Allspice tea and allspice infusion can be consumed for this purpose.

Chills

Allspice is used to manage chills since it has a warming effect and increases the circulation of blood. Allspice tea and allspice infusion can be consumed for this purpose. Allspice salve can be massaged on the hands for this purpose.

High blood pressure

Allspice is given to persons with hypertension or high blood pressure.

Diabetes

Allspice is taken by persons with diabetes.

Obesity

Allspice is taken by person who are obese or overweight.

Toothache

Allspice oil is applied to the teeth to relieve toothaches.

3

SAFETY PRECAUTIONS

1. Allspice contains a chemical known as eugenol which can slow the clotting of blood and increase the chance of bleeding excessively during or after surgery. It should therefore not be used 2 weeks before surgery.

2. Persons with stomach ulcers, ulcerative colitis, and diverticulitis should avoid eating food with allspice.

3. Hypersensitive individuals can develop serious allergic reactions if they consume dishes with excess allspice. They may also develop gastrointestinal irritation, central nervous system depression and seizures.

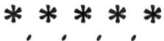

4

DRUG INTERACTIONS

Allspice should not be used together with medications like anticoagulants and antiplatelet drugs which slow the clotting of blood since it can increase the chances of bleeding. Examples of these medications include aspirin, clopidogrel (Plavix), diclofenac (Voltaren), ibuprofen (Advil), naproxen (Naprosyn), dalteparin (Fragmin), enoxaparin, (Lovenox), heparin, warfarin (Coumadin).

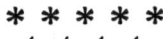

5

COOKING TIPS

Flavor

Fragrantly spicy

Goes well with

Savory meat dishes made with beef, lamb and wild game. Also used in curry recipes. It is also used in sweet dishes like fruit pies, puddings, cakes and chocolate.

Can be substituted with

Cinnamon and cloves mixture

Tips

Allspice can inhibit the activity of yeast.

6 whole allspice berries are equivalent to ½ teaspoon of allspice powder.

When used for cooking, allspice should be added at the final stages since prolonged cooking results in evaporation of the healing aromatic oils.

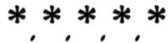

6

HERBAL RECIPES

Allspice Tea

Equipment

Kettle

Tea cup

***

Ingredients

1 teaspoon of allspice powder

1 cup of boiling water

Honey to taste (optional)

***

Instructions

1. Put the allspice in a tea cup, add the boiling water and let it steep while covered for 10 -15 minutes.

3. Add honey (if using) to suit your taste before drinking.

***

Tips

Allspice tea can be taken twice a day between meals to relieve flatulence.

*****

Allspice Decoction

Equipment
Non-reactive heavy saucepan

***

Ingredients
1 oz (30 grams) herb

1 pint (500 ml) water

***

Instructions
1. Place the allspice and water in the saucepan, cover it and slowly bring the mixture to a simmering boil for 20 minutes.

2. Remove from the heat source and let the mixture cool to drinking temperature.

3. Strain the mixture, measure it and pour the liquid into a clean saucepan.

4. Heat the liquid until it begins to steam. Reduce the heat and let the liquid continue to steam until it is reduced to half its original volume. This may take 45 minutes to 1 hour.

5. Pour the decoction into a clean bottle.

***

Tips
1. Store the decoction in the refrigerator to lengthen its life.

*****

Allspice Poultice

Equipment

Cheesecloth or old cotton sheet strips

***

Ingredients

1 tablespoon powdered allspice

Boiling water

***

Instructions

1. Add enough boiling water to the allspice to wet it and make a thick paste.

2. Spoon the herb paste onto the cheesecloth (or bed sheet strips) to make the poultice.

3. To use, apply the poultice to the affected area and cover with another piece of hot, wet cloth. Replace the hot, wet cloth when it cools with another hot one to keep the poultice hot.

*****

Allspice Tincture

Equipment

Glass jar with tight fitting lid

Dark tincture bottles

Cheesecloth

Labels

***

Ingredients

7 oz (200 gm) of allspice powder

30 oz (1 liter) of 80-100 proof vodka

***

Instructions

1. Fill 1/3 of the glass jar with the allspice.

2. Add the vodka to completely fill the jar to the top.

3. Seal the jar and label it with the date of preparation and name of herb used.

4. Store the glass jar in a dark place for 6 weeks ensuring that you shake them weekly.

5. After 6 weeks strain out the herbs with a cheesecloth and pour the tincture into dark tincture bottles.

6. Label the tincture bottles with the date and name of herb used.

7. Store your herbal tinctures away from light and heat.

***

Tips

1. Pick your herbs early in the morning just after the dew has dried.

2. You can leave the herbs in the alcohol for up to 6 months if you want to create very strong tinctures.

3. To make your tinctures doubly strong, you can pour the tincture after straining in step 5 above and store it for six more weeks.

4. Though the dose varies, a standard dose is 1 teaspoon diluted in water or tea and taken 1-3 times a day.

*****

Allspice Infused Oil

Equipment

Double boiler

Large glass bowl

Sieve and cheesecloth

Sterilized dark jars

***

Ingredients

16 fl oz. (500 ml) pure vegetable oil such as sweet almond oil or sunflower oil

8 oz. (250 grams) allspice powder

***

Instructions

1. Place the allspice and oil in the glass bowl ensuring that the oil covers the spice. Simmer them in a double boiler for one hour at a temperature of around 120 degrees Fahrenheit (49 degrees Celsius). Do not let the oil and herbs boil. You can repeat this step several times after letting the oils cool to create more concentrated herb infused oils. You can make your oils even more concentrated by adding a fresh bunch of herbs with each re-simmering.

2. Strain the mixture through the sieve and cheesecloth into a clean, dark jar ensuring you squeeze out as much oil as you can from the spice in the cheesecloth.

3. Label your jars with the manufacturing date, expiry date, herb and oils used.

4. Store your allspice infused oils in a cool dark place or in the refrigerator and use them within 3 months.

*****

Allspice Salve

Equipment
Double boiler

Large glass bowl

Sterilized dark jars or tins

***

Ingredients
8 oz. (250 ml or 1 cup) herb infused vegetable oil (see previous recipe)

1 oz. (30 grams) beeswax

50 drops (2.5 ml or ½ teaspoon) essential oils like lavender essential oil

***

Instructions
1. Place the beeswax and allspice infused oil in the glass bowl and melt them in a double boiler.

2. Once melted remove from the heat source and add the essential oil.

3. Pour the melted oils into the storage jars or tins and allow to cool completely.

4. Store the salves in a cool dark place.

***

Tips
1. When making a salve to treat arthritis use eucalyptus, peppermint or lavender essential oil.

2. When making a salve to treat muscle aches use Roman chamomile, marjoram or lavender essential oil.

3. When making a salve to treat coughs and colds use eucalyptus, lemon or peppermint essential oil.

*****

Allspice Syrup

Equipment

Saucepan

Jar with airtight lid

***

Ingredients

1 quart (1000 ml) filtered water

1 cup allspice powder

1 cup honey

***

Instructions

1. Place the water and allspice in a saucepan and bring to a boil.

2. Reduce the heat and let it simmer while it is partially covered until the volume is reduced to half the original volume.

3. Strain the mixture through a sieve or cheesecloth to remove the herbs.

4. Measure 1 pint (500 mls) of the liquid and add the honey.

5. Cook for a few minutes as you stir it so that it thickens.

6. Store the syrup in an airtight container in the fridge for up to 2 months.

###

ABOUT THE AUTHOR

Marian Kim is an experienced alternative medicine practitioner.

OTHER BOOKS BY THE AUTHOR

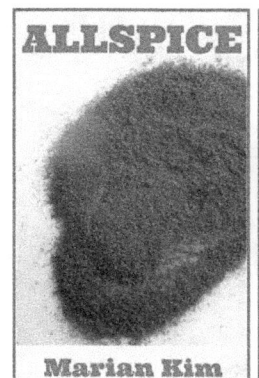

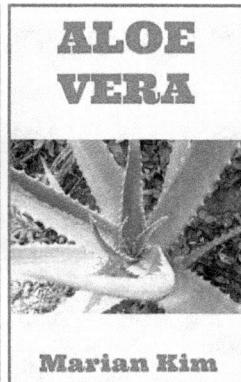

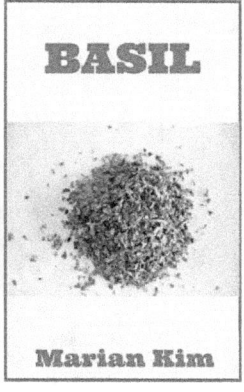

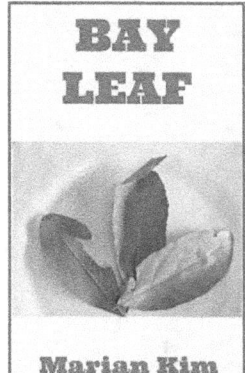

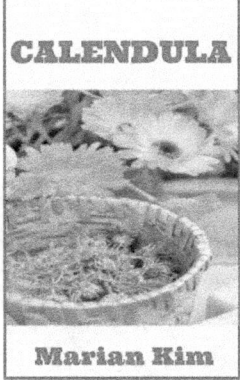

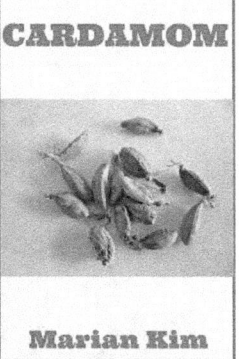

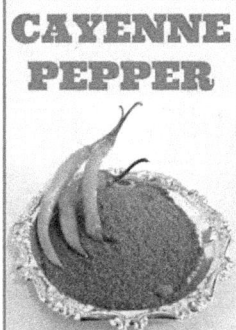

CAYENNE PEPPER

Marian Kim

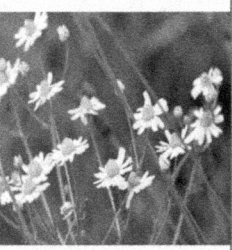

CHAMOMILE

Marian Kim

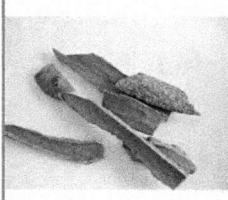

CILANTRO & CORIANDER

Marian Kim

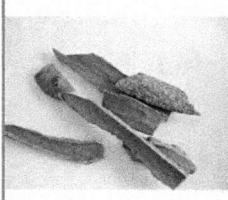

CINNAMON

Marian Kim

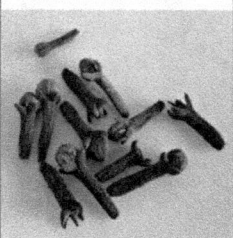

CLOVES

Marian Kim

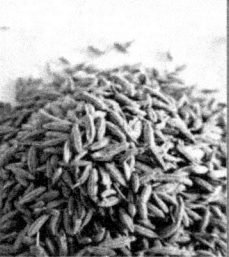

CUMIN

Marian Kim

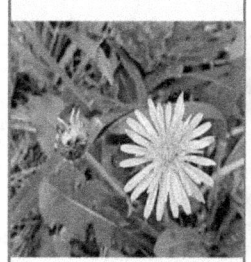

DANDELION

Marian Kim

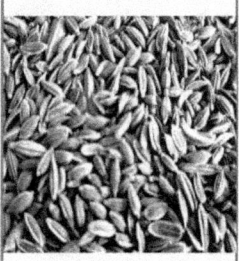

DILL

Marian Kim

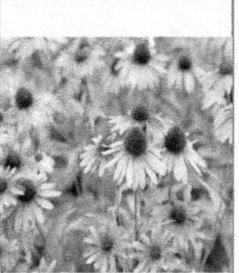

ECHINACEA

Marian Kim

FENNEL

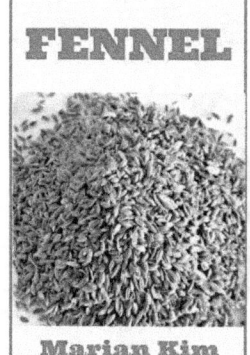

Marian Kim

FENUGREEK

Marian Kim

GARLIC

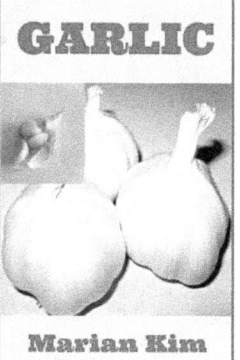

Marian Kim

GINGER

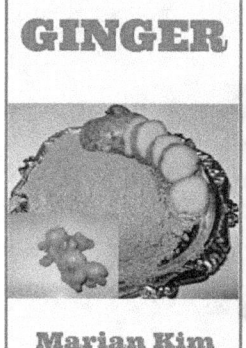

Marian Kim

GINKGO BILOBA

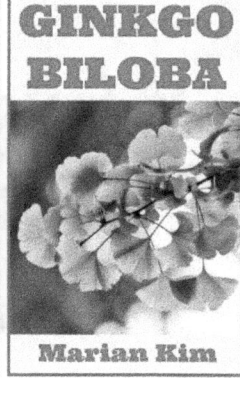

Marian Kim

GINSENG

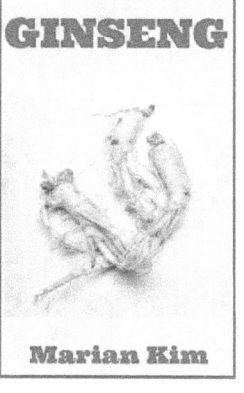

Marian Kim

LAVENDER

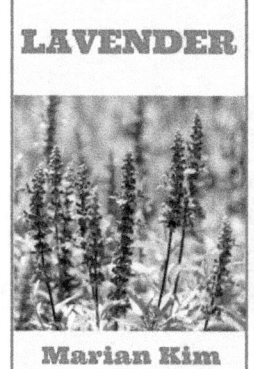

Marian Kim

MUSTARD

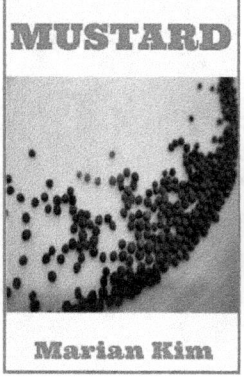

Marian Kim

NEEM

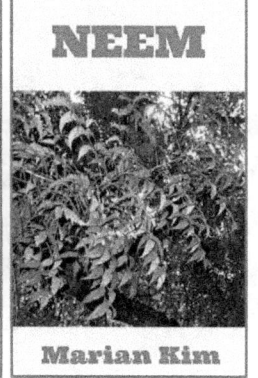

Marian Kim

NUTMEG & MACE

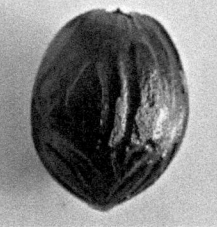

Marian Kim

OREGANO

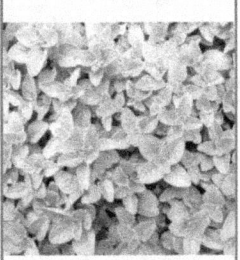

Marian Kim

PAPRIKA

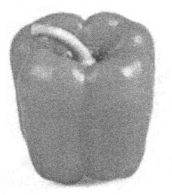

Marian Kim

PARSLEY

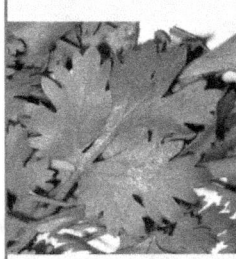

Marian Kim

BLACK & WHITE PEPPER

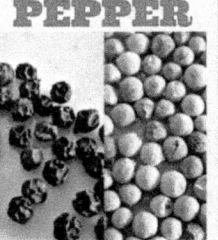

Marian Kim

PEPPERMINT

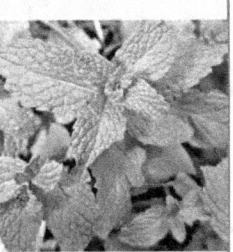

Marian Kim

ROSE HIPS

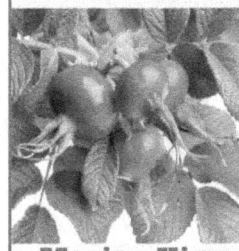

Marian Kim

ROSE PETALS

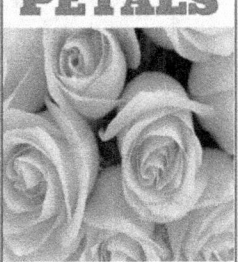

Marian Kim

ROSEMARY

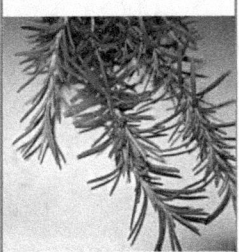

Marian Kim

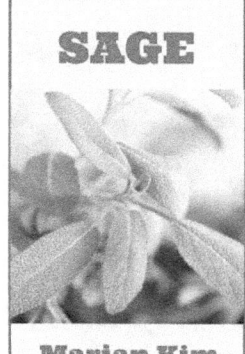

SAGE

Marian Kim

ST. JOHN'S WORT

Marian Kim

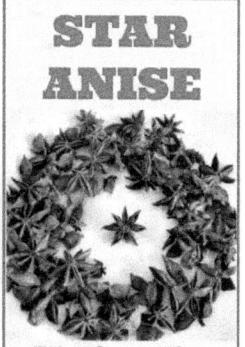

STAR ANISE

Marian Kim

STINGING NETTLE

Marian Kim

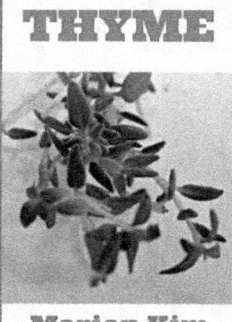

THYME

Marian Kim

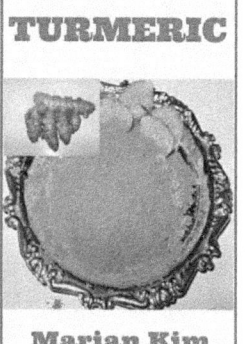

TURMERIC

Marian Kim

WITCH HAZEL

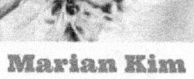

Marian Kim

YARROW

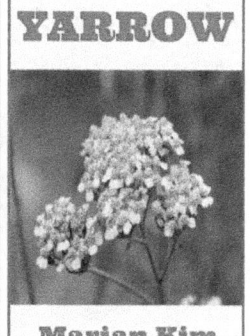

Marian Kim

*****